How to Handle Emotional stress

Tips for coping with stress and healthy living

By Sarah k.Moore

Table of content

Chapter 1:What is emotional stress?

Stresses typically faced nowadays include pressure at job, studies, health concerns, social circumstances, finances, future planning, and career decisions, among others.

Stress is emotional tension or a form of mental distress that many of us encounter in our modern day, hectic lifestyles. However, according to specialists, not all stress results from unfavorable events. Occasionally, even excellent news may lead to unexpected tension and stress as a result of our overthinking about the outcome of such news. What's more, in tiny doses, stress can even help us perform better and get things done on time, but some types of stress can also bring about life-threatening difficulties.

The sense of psychological tension and anxiety created by situations of danger, threat, and loss of personal security or by internal conflicts, frustrations, loss of self-esteem, and sadness.

Emotional stress itself can be tough to deal with and can make patients feel wretched, hurt, and uncomfortable - and it's a sort of stress that gives no special benefits.

Given that stress has been connected as a cofactor in 95% of all disease processes, understanding how to properly manage stress is a cornerstone of holistic, alternative health, and healing.

This learning process begins with recognizing or identifying four particular types of stress affecting you and how these stressors (that is, what demands a change from you) are showing up or manifesting as symptoms in your life.

Stress factors broadly divide into four forms or categories: physical stress, psychological stress, psychosocial stress, and psychospiritual stress.

Physical stress: trauma (injury, infection, surgery), intense physical labor/over-exertion, environmental pollution (pesticides, herbicides, toxins, heavy metals, inadequate light, radiation, noise, electromagnetic fields), illness (viral, bacterial, or fungal agents), fatigue, inadequate oxygen supply, hypoglycemia (low blood sugar), hormonal and/or biochemical imbalances, dietary stress (nutritional deficiencies, food allergies and sensitivities, unhealthy eating habits), dehydration, substance abuse, dental challenges, and musculoskeletal misalignments/imbalances.

Psychological stress: emotional stress (resentments, fears, frustration, sadness, anger, grief/bereavement), cognitive stress (information overload, accelerated sense of time, worry, guilt, shame, jealousy, resistance, attachments, self-criticism, self-loathing, unworkable perfectionism, anxiety, panic attacks, not feeling like yourself, not feeling like things are real, and a sense of being out of control/not being in control), and perceptual stress (beliefs, roles, stories, attitudes, worldview) (beliefs, roles, stories, attitudes, worldview).

Psychosocial stress: relationship/marriage troubles (partner, siblings, children, family, employer, co-workers, employer), lack of social support, lack of resources for proper survival, loss of employment/investments/savings, loss of loved ones, bankruptcy, house foreclosure, and isolation

Psycho-spiritual stress: a crisis of values, meaning, and purpose; joyless striving (instead of productive, enjoyable, meaningful, and rewarding employment); and a misalignment with one's underlying spiritual convictions.

Overall, badly or ineffectively managed stress usually takes a toll on the body. When stress-related feelings, moods, and emotions are pushed into the body, the soma, this is usually termed psychosomatic or psychogenic illness, including headaches, heart palpitations, physical/cognitive/emotional pain and suffering, constricted throat and shallow, constricted breathing, clammy palms, fatigue, nausea, anxiety, allergies, asthma, autoimmune syndromes related to an ineffective functioning of the immune system, hypertension (high blood pressure), and gastrointestinal disturbances such as diarrhea, upset stomach, duodenal ulcers, and esophageal reflux syndrome.

Prolonged stress can result in reduced immune function, increased vulnerability to infectious and immunological-related illnesses, and cancer. Emotional stress can also result in hormone abnormalities (adrenal, pituitary, thyroid, etcetera) that further interfere with optimal immune functioning.

Cognitive: nervous thoughts, frightened anticipation, poor attention, difficulties with remembering.

Emotional: emotions of tension, irritation, restlessness, concern, inability to relax, depression.

Behavioral: task avoidance; sleep troubles; difficulty completing work assignments; fidgeting; tremors; strained face; clenched fists; sobbing; changes in drinking, eating, or smoking habits.

Physiological: Stiff or tense muscles, grinding teeth, sweating, faint feelings, choking feelings, difficulty in swallowing, stomachache, nausea, vomiting, loosening of bowels, constipation, frequency and urgency of urination, loss of interest in sex, tiredness, shakiness or tremors, weight loss or gain, awareness of heart beat.

Social: Some people, amid stressful situations, tend to seek out others to be around. Other folks withdraw under stress. Also, the quality of relationships might change when a person is under stress.

Chapter 2:Symptoms of mental stress?

The physical indications of stress include difficulties with the cardiovascular system, digestive system, immunological system, endocrine system, muscular system, reproductive system, and respiratory system. The emotional indications of stress are irritability or moodiness, anxiety, depression, feeling overwhelmed or unmotivated, and loneliness and isolation.

The physical indications of stress include difficulties with the cardiovascular system, digestive system, immunological system, endocrine system, muscular system, reproductive system, and respiratory system. The emotional indications of stress are irritability or moodiness, anxiety, depression, feeling overwhelmed or unmotivated, and loneliness and isolation.

Stress is a feeling of emotional or physical tension; it's a natural reaction to a threat, demand, or difficulty. Your body reacts to these stimuli with physical and emotional responses.

Stress can have a range of effects on our behavior and emotions. Stress also affects many systems, organs, and tissues all throughout the body.

Signs and symptoms of stress

Stress affects the entire body, generating broad physical effects. Stress expresses physically in these body systems:

Cardiovascular system

Stress often pushes your body into a "fight or flight" response, in which stress hormones like adrenaline, noradrenaline, and cortisol cause your heart rate to accelerate. Stress creates greater contractions of the heart muscle. Also, the blood arteries that direct blood to the major muscles and the heart widen, which elevates your blood pressure, increasing your risk of suffering a heart attack or stroke.

Digestive system

When you're anxious, your liver will generate additional blood sugar (glucose) to improve your energy. This flood of blood sugar over time may increase your risk of getting type 2 diabetes.

Your digestive tract may also encounter trouble from a rush of stress hormones, fast breathing, and increased heart rate. You may have constipation, diarrhea, heartburn or acid reflux, cramping or stomach pain, and even nausea and vomiting.

immune system

Over time, stress chemicals can impair your immune system. If you're constantly stressed, you're more prone to viral diseases and other infections.

Endocrine system

When your brain recognizes a threat, it sets off a cascade of processes involving the hypothalamic-pituitary-adrenal (HPA) axis. This leads to an acceleration in the synthesis of steroid hormones—including cortisol, which is recognized as the principal stress hormone.

muscular system

When you're stressed, your muscles may stiffen up. Though muscles generally relax when your stress levels go down, chronically stressed individuals may be tense all the time.

Reproductive system

Acute stress may cause males to create more testosterone. However, continuous stress can induce a drop in testosterone, which may cause erectile dysfunction or lower sperm production. Chronic stress may also raise the risk of infection in male reproductive organs.

Stress can alter women's menstrual cycles in the form of heavier, irregular, or more painful periods. Chronic stress may also increase symptoms of menopause. Stress can disrupt the pregnancy process, including challenges to conceive.

Respiratory system

If you're facing stress, you'll likely breathe quicker. This occurs because your body is seeking to quickly circulate oxygen-rich blood throughout your body. If you already have a breathing issue like asthma, you may struggle to tolerate the increased lung exertion.

Emotional indications of stress

Chronic stress can create a variety of emotional symptoms and damage your general well-being and mental health. Emotional signs of chronic stress can include:

- Irritability or moodiness.

- Anxiety

- Depression

- Feeling overwhelmed or unmotivated?

- Loneliness and solitude

Causes of stress

Situations and events that create stress are known as stressors, which are external causes. Stress can also be induced by internal causes, such as how you view and interpret your life.

Common external causes of stress are:

- Your job or schoolwork

- Your relationships and family.

- Your finances

- Your living situation

- Your schedule

Common internal sources of stress are:

Lack of flexibility or rigid thinking

Negative self-talk or low self-esteem

Negativity, or pessimism,

Perfectionism

Desire for control or incapacity to accept uncertainty

It is vital to recognize that stressors vary amongst persons. A difficult circumstance for one individual could be a joyful or exhilarating event for another person.

When to see the doctor for stress

Over time, stress can have a severe influence on your physical or mental health. If you have attempted to manage your stress on your own but are still struggling, reach out to your doctor. They may be able to offer more skills or recommend you to a mental health counselor for more support.

Call your doctor immediately if your stress is causing you to develop suicidal thoughts or use drugs or alcohol more regularly. They can provide tools and guidance to help you manage your stress.

Stress diagnosis

Stress is considered a breakdown of normal homeostasis. Under stress, your body responds physiologically to increased activity of both the hypothalamic-pituitary-adrenal (HPA) axis and the sympathoadrenal system (SAS) . This means that a diagnosis depends on a multiplicity of circumstances and is complex. Diagnostic tools may include questionnaires, biochemical tests, and physiologic procedures.

Chapter 3:Chronic stress symptoms?

Stress is a biological response to demanding situations. It causes the body to release hormones, such as cortisol and adrenaline.

These hormones help prepare the body to take action, for example, by increasing the heart and breath rates. When this occurs, a doctor might describe a person as being in a state of heightened alertness or arousal.

Many factors can trigger a stress response, including dangerous situations and psychological pressures, such as work deadlines, exams, and sporting events.

The physical effects of stress usually do not last long. However, some people find themselves in a nearly constant state of heightened alertness. This is chronic stress.

Some potential causes of chronic stress include:

- high-pressure jobs
- financial difficulties
- challenging relationships

Chronic stress puts pressure on the body for an extended period. This can cause a range of symptoms and increase the risk of developing certain illnesses.

Chronic stress affects the whole body. It can have several physical or psychological symptoms, which can make functioning on a daily basis more challenging.

The type and severity of symptoms vary considerably from person to person.

Signs and symptoms of chronic stress can include:

Irritability, which can be extreme:
- fatigue
- headaches
- Difficulty concentrating, or an inability to do so
- Rapid, disorganized thoughts
- Difficulty sleeping
- Digestive problems
- changes in appetite
- feeling helpless
- A perceived loss of control
- low self-esteem
- loss of sexual desire

- Nervousness
- frequent infections or illnesses

Examples of stress

A variety of life experiences can cause stress, and these may begin in childhood. When children experience traumatic events, it can lead to the development of chronic stress that may last into adulthood.

These types of events are known as adverse childhood experiences (ACEs). In research by the Centers for Disease Control and Prevention (CDC), 61% of adults surveyed across 25 states said they had experienced at least one type of ACE, and nearly 1 in 6 had experienced four or more types.

Examples of ACEs include:

mental illness in one or more parents
emotional, physical, or sexual abuse
substance misuse in the family
parental divorce
homelessness
incarceration of a parent or close family member
In adulthood, chronic stress can happen as a result of very similar causes, as well as:

- problems in the workplace

- unemployment or financial problems
- injury that impacts a person's daily life
- concern about problems in the country or the world

According to the Stress in America 2020 survey by the American Psychological Association (APA), 65% of people surveyed said the current uncertainty in the nation is stressful, and 60% are overwhelmed by the issues the country is facing.

In addition, 70% of parents reported family responsibilities as a source of stress, and 63% are stressed by the impact of COVID-19 on the 2019-20 school year.

Chronic stress can also affect historically marginalized groups differently than others. In 2019, surveys showed that Black and Hispanic people are three timesTrusted Source more likely to be stressed by lack of food and safe housing, discrimination, and health inequities.

More recently, the APA also reported that nearly three-quarters of Black adults (74%), 60% of Hispanic adults, and 65% of white adults said the Capitol breach in 2020 caused them a lot of stress.

Treatment

If strategies such as those listed above are not helping, it is important to see a healthcare professional for advice and support. A doctor may recommend psychological therapy, such as cognitive behavioral therapy (CBT).

One established aim of CBT is to help people deal with chronic stress. In structured sessions, a therapist works to enable a person to modify their behaviors, thoughts, and feelings concerning stressors.

CBT can also help a person develop tools and coping mechanisms to manage stress responses.

Sometimes, a doctor recommends medications to help treat some symptoms of chronic stress. For example, they may prescribe antidepressants to treat anxiety or depression. For people with trouble sleeping, doctors may prescribe sedatives.

Health effects

Research has shown that chronic stress can impact the brain and the immune system. The brain's neural networks, especially in the prefrontal cortex (PFC), can actually reduce in size. Doctors have seen this in imaging of people's brains. When this happens, it may lead to cognitive, emotional, and behavioral dysfunctions.

When a person experiences stress, this stimulates their immune system to react. Over time, when stress is chronic, the immune system can become overstimulated. This may lead to the development of diseases and health problems.

Over long periods, chronic stress can contribute to the development of a range of physical and mental disorders, including:

- heart disease
- high blood pressure
- Diabetes
- obesity
- A weakened immune system
- sexual dysfunction
- Gastrointestinal disorders
- skin irritation
- Respiratory infections
- Autoimmune diseases
- Insomnia
- Burnout
- Depression
- Anxiety disorders
- post-traumatic stress disorder (PTSD)
- schizophrenia

Chronic stress vs. acute stress

Generally, acute stress is stress that a person experiences short-term. Acute stress typically manifests immediately after a person experiences a stressor as a fight-or-flight reaction.

An acute stress disorder is more serious and typically occurs in the first month after a person experiences trauma. This is similar to post-traumatic stress disorder (PTSD), but a person cannot have a diagnosis of PTSD until they have experienced symptoms for longer than a month.

Stress can also be episodic, which means a person experiences it over a long time but inconsistently. They experience stressful periods and periods with less or no stress. In comparison, chronic stress is stress that a person experiences continuously throughout their life to the point where feeling stressed becomes a normal state of being.

Managing stress
Chronic stress can seem overwhelming, and a person may feel unable to regain control over their life.

However, a number of strategies can help to reduce stress levels and improve well-being.

Some methods for managing stress include:

Understanding the signs and symptoms. These indications vary, but if a person can recognize their own signals of stress, they will be better able to manage them. Speaking to friends and family. They can provide emotional support and the motivation to take action.

Identifying triggers. It is not always possible to avoid triggers of stress. However, taking note of specific triggers can help a person to develop coping and management strategies, which may involve reducing exposure.

Exercising regularly. Physical activity increases the body's production of endorphins, which are chemicals that boost the mood and reduce stress. Exercise can involve walking, cycling, running, working out, or playing sports.

Trying mindfulness. People who practice this form of meditation use breathing and thought techniques to create an awareness of their body and surroundings.

Research suggests that mindfulness can have a positive impact on stress, anxiety, and depression.

Improving sleep quality. Getting too little sleep or sleep of poor quality can contribute to stress. Try to get at least 7 hours every night, and set regular times for going to sleep and waking up. Avoid caffeine, eating, and intense physical activity in the hours before bed.

It can also help to unwind before sleeping by listening to music, reading a book, taking a warm bath, or meditating, for example.

When to see a doctor

Do not try to deal with chronic stress alone. If self-help strategies are not working, a doctor can provide support and advice about treatment options. They can also refer a person to a more specialized healthcare provider, such as a psychologist or psychiatrist.

Anyone feeling overwhelmed by stress should see a doctor as soon as possible, especially if they are having suicidal thoughts or using drugs or alcohol to cope.

Recovery

Strategies to recover from chronic stress can include practicing mindfulness activities such as meditation and breathing exercises. People can also have a support system composed of family and friends, as well as a counselor or a psychiatrist if needed.

A psychiatrist can prescribe medication to reduce stress. A counselor can help a person explore the causes of their stress in order to recognize them and find a healthy coping mechanism. The earlier a person seeks help or treatment, the quicker their recovery may be.

Takeaway

Stress is a regular part of daily life. Short-lived stress is generally harmless, but when it lasts and becomes chronic, it can cause a range of symptoms. It can also contribute to the development of physical and mental disorders.

Self-help techniques include identifying triggers, developing coping and avoidance strategies, reaching out to friends and family, and practicing mindfulness.

If these techniques are not working, or if stress is becoming overwhelming, a person should speak to a healthcare professional.

Many people have chronic stress and anxiety. They face symptoms such as nervousness, agitation, tension, a racing heart, and chest pain.

In fact, anxiety is among the most common mental health issues. In the United States, more than 18 percent of adults are affected by anxiety disorders each year.

In some cases, another health condition, such as an overactive thyroid, can lead to an anxiety disorder. Getting an accurate diagnosis can ensure that a person receives the best treatment.

However, alterations to the diet and some natural supplements can change the way anti anxiety medications work, so it is essential to consult a doctor before trying these solutions. The doctor may also be able to recommend other natural remedies.

1. Exercise
Exercise may help to treat anxiety.
Exercise is a great way to burn off anxious energy, and research tends to support this use.

For example, a 2015 review of 12 randomized controlled trials found that exercise may be a treatment for anxiety. However, the review cautioned that only research of higher quality could determine how effective it is.

Exercise may also help with anxiety caused by stressful circumstances. Results of a 2016 study, for example, suggest that exercise can benefit people with anxiety related to quitting smoking.

2. Meditation
Meditation can help to slow racing thoughts, making it easier to manage stress and anxiety. A wide range of meditation styles, including mindfulness and meditation during yoga, may help.

Mindfulness-based meditation is increasingly popular in therapy. A 2010 meta-analytic review suggests that it can be highly effective for people with disorders relating to mood and anxiety.

3. Relaxation exercises

Some people unconsciously tense the muscles and clench the jaw in response to anxiety. Progressive relaxation exercises can help.

Try lying in a comfortable position and slowly constricting and relaxing each muscle group, beginning with the toes and working up to the shoulders and jaw.

4. Writing

Finding a way to express anxiety can make it feel more manageable.

Some research suggests that journaling and other forms of writing can help people to cope better with anxiety.

A 2016 study, for example, found that creative writing may help children and teens to manage anxiety.

5. Time management strategies

Some people feel anxious if they have too many commitments at once. These may involve family, work, and health-related activities. Having a plan in place for the next necessary action can help to keep this anxiety at bay.

Effective time management strategies can help people to focus on one task at a time. Book-based planners and online calendars can help, as can resisting the urge to multitask.

Some people find that breaking major projects down into manageable steps can help them to accomplish those tasks with less stress.

6. Aromatherapy
Smelling soothing plant oils can help to ease stress and anxiety. Certain scents work better for some people than others, so consider experimenting with various options.

Lavender may be especially helpful. A 2012 study tested the effects of aromatherapy with lavender on insomnia in 67 women aged 45–55. Results suggest that the aromatherapy may reduce the heart rate in the short term and help to ease sleep issues in the long term.

7. Cannabidiol oil
CBD oil comes from the marijuana plant.
Cannabidiol (CBD) oil is a derivative of the cannabis, or marijuana, plant.

Unlike other forms of marijuana, CBD oil does not contain tetrahydrocannabinol, or THC, which is the substance that creates a "high."

CBD oil is readily available without a prescription in many alternative healthcare shops. Preliminary research suggests that it has significant potential to reduce anxiety and panic.

In areas where medical marijuana is legal, doctors may also be able to prescribe the oil.

8. Herbal teas
Many herbal teas promise to help with anxiety and ease sleep.

Some people find the process of making and drinking tea soothing, but some teas may have a more direct effect on the brain that results in reduced anxiety.

Results of a small 2018 trial suggest that chamomile can alter levels of cortisol, a stress hormone.

9. Herbal supplements
Like herbal teas, many herbal supplements claim to reduce anxiety. However, little scientific evidence supports these claims.

It is vital to work with a doctor who is knowledgeable about herbal supplements and their potential interactions with other drugs.

10. Time with animals
Pets offer companionship, love, and support. Research published in 2018 confirmed that pets can be beneficial to people with a variety of mental health issues, including anxiety.

While many people prefer cats, dogs, and other small mammals, people with allergies will be pleased to learn that the pet does have to be furry to provide support.

A 2015 study found that caring for crickets could improve psychological health in older people.

Spending time with animals can also reduce anxiety and stress associated with trauma. Results of a 2015 systematic review suggest that grooming and spending time with horses can alleviate some of these effects.

Other treatment options
Therapy may help to treat chronic anxiety.
Anxiety that is chronic or interferes with a person's ability to function warrants treatment.

When there is no underlying medical condition, such as a thyroid problem, therapy is the most popular form of treatment.

Therapy can help a person to understand what triggers their anxiety. It can also help with making positive lifestyle changes and working through trauma.

One of the most effective therapies for anxiety is called cognitive behavioral therapy (CBT). The goal is to help a person understand how their thoughts affect their emotions and behavior and to replace those reactions with positive or constructive alternatives.

CBT can help with generalized anxiety and anxiety relating to a specific issue, such as work or an instance of trauma.

Medication can also help a person to manage chronic anxiety. A doctor may prescribe medications in any of the following groups:

antianxiety drugs called benzodiazepines, including Xanax and Valium
antidepressants called selective serotonin reuptake inhibitors, including Prozac
sleeping medications, if anxiety interferes with sleep

People should follow the doctor's instructions when using these drugs, as they can have severe and possibly life threatening adverse effects.

Natural anxiety remedies can replace or complement traditional treatments.

Outlook
Untreated anxiety can get worse and cause more stress in a person's life. However, anxiety is highly treatable with therapy, natural remedies, lifestyle changes, and medications.

A person may need to try several combinations of therapies and remedies before finding one that works. A doctor can help a person to determine which options are best.

Chapter 4:Causes of mental stress?

Stress is normal and, to some extent, an essential component of life. Despite it being something everyone experiences, what causes stress might differ from person to person.

For instance, one person may become irritated and overwhelmed by a significant traffic delay, while another might turn up their music and consider it a slight annoyance. A dispute with a friend can follow one person around for the remainder of the day, while another might effortlessly brush it off.

What's causing you stress may already be something you're abundantly aware of. But considering the significance of keeping stress in check when it comes to reducing the effects it can have on your physical and mental health, it's worth opening yourself up to the potential that other factors may be at play, too. Craft your stress-reduction plan with all of them in mind.

Financial Problems

According to the American Psychological Association (APA), money is the main source of stress in the United States. In a 2015 poll, the APA stated that 72% of Americans fretted about money at least some of the time over the preceding month. 1 The majority of the survey participants rated money as being a substantial source of stress, with 77% feeling considerable anxiety about finances.

Signs of financial stress may include:

- Arguing with loved ones regarding money

- Being frightened to open the mail or answer the phone

- Feeling guilty because you spent money on non-essentials

- Worrying and feeling nervous about money

In the long term, stress related to finances leads to distress, which may raise blood pressure and produce headaches, upset stomach, chest pain, insomnia, and an overall sensation of sickness. Financial stress has also been related to a number of health concerns, including depression, anxiety, skin disorders, diabetes, and arthritis.

According to the Centers for Disease Control and Prevention (CDC), Americans today spend 8% more time at work compared to 20 years ago, and about 13% of adults work a second job. At least 40% report their employment is demanding, and 26% report they often feel burned out by their work. 2

Any variety of causes can contribute to workplace stress, including too much work, job insecurity, dissatisfaction with a job or career, and disagreements with a boss and/or co-workers.

Whether you are anxious about a specific project or feeling unfairly treated, putting your job ahead of everything else can damage many parts of your life, including personal relationships and mental and physical health.

Factors outside of the job itself also play an influence in work stress, including a person's psychological make-up, general health, and personal life. and the amount of emotional support they have outside of work.

The indicators of work-related stress might be physical or psychological, including:

- Anxiety

- Depression

- Difficulty concentrating or making decisions

- Fatigue

- Headache

- Heart palpitations

- Mood swings

- Muscle tightness and discomfort

- Stomach troubles

Should You Tell Your Boss If You Have a Mental Health Condition?

Some people may feel overwhelmed and struggle to manage, which might affect their behavior as well. Job stress may encourage people to have:

- Diminished creativity and initiative

- Disinterest

- Decline in work performance.

- Increased sick days

- Isolation

- Lower levels of patience and increasing levels of frustration

- Problems with personal connections

Personal Relationships.

There are people in all of our lives that give us stress. It could be a family member, an intimate partner, a friend, or co-worker. Toxic people lurk in all corners of our life, and the stress we encounter from these connections can impair our physical and emotional health.

There are several causes of stress in love relationships, and when couples are always under strain, the relationship could be at the risk of failing.

Common relationship stressors include:

- being too busy to spend time with each other and share duties.

- Intimacy and sex have become infrequent due to workload, health concerns, and any number of other reasons.

- There is abuse or control in the relationship

- You and your lover are not communicating.

- You and/or your spouse are consuming too much alcohol and/or taking drugs.

- You or your partner are thinking about divorce.

The signals of stress related to personal relationships are comparable to normal symptoms of general stress and may include physical health problems, sleep problems, sadness, and anxiety.

You may also find yourself avoiding or having confrontation with the individual, or getting easily irritated by their presence.

Sometimes, personal relationship stress can also be tied to our relationships with others on social media platforms, such as Facebook. For example, social media tends to automatically encourage comparing yourself to others, which can contribute to the stress of feeling inadequate. It also makes bullying simpler.

Parenting

Parents are often challenged with managing busy schedules that involve work, domestic obligations, and raising children. These demands result in parenting stress.

High levels of parenting stress can drive a parent to be harsh, negative, and authoritarian in their relationships with their children. Parenting stress can also reduce the quality of parent-child connections. For example, you may not have open communication, so your child doesn't turn to you for guidance or you and your child may argue constantly.

Sources of parenting stress may include being low-income, working long hours, single parenting, marital or relationship problems, or having a child who has been diagnosed with a behavioral condition or developmental handicap.

Parents of children with behavior issues and developmental impairments have the highest risk for parenting stress. In fact, multiple studies suggest parents of children with autism spectrum disorder report higher levels of parenting stress than families whose children do not have the illness. 7

Daily Life and Busyness

Day-to-day pressures are our daily hassles. They include problems like misplacing keys, running late, and forgetting to carry a crucial item with you when leaving the house. Usually, they are simply minor setbacks, but if they become frequent, they become a source of concern, impacting physical and/or psychological health.

The stress of being overly busy is becoming more and more widespread. These days, people are busier than ever, and it adds a lot of stress to their life.

In some circumstances, busyness is due to need, such as having to work a second job. Other times, it is due to guilt and not wanting to disappoint others. People may not say "no" and wind up having little time for themselves, or they may disregard their own basic needs, such as eating correctly and exercising, due to a lack of time.

How to Say "No"

Perception and Resources

Your personality qualities and the resources you have available to you tie into all of the above and can be independent sources of stress as well.

Extroverts, for example, tend to encounter less stress in daily life and have better social resources, which buffer against stress. Perfectionists, on the other hand, may excessively stress themselves owing to their stringent standards, experiencing more negative mental and physical health consequences than those who just focus on high success.

Those who are "type A" can worry everyone around them, even themselves. Those with enough money to employ help can delegate onerous jobs, thus this resource can provide an edge over those who struggle to make ends meet and must work harder to save cash.

Chapter 5:How to deal with emotional stress

Dealing with Emotional Stress:

Though recovering from a stressful situation may not be easy, emotional stress can certainly be managed and reduced. Here are a few ways that can help you effectively cope with emotional stress:

Accept Things for What They Are: Thinking you can control everything around you is unrealistic and only leads to more stress. Accept the fact that things don't always go as planned, that there are certain situations over which you have no control. Learning to accept certain things for what they are is vital to reducing emotional stress levels.

Distract Yourself from Emotional Pain: Many people advocate sharing painful and unpleasant experiences as a way of coping with emotional pain – and most of us have done so with mixed results. To some extent, this advice holds true as bottling up emotions can have serious consequences on a person's mental, and sometimes even physical, health. However, studies have shown that distracting yourself from emotional pain and engaging in emotionally healthier activities is a better way of dealing with emotional stress. You can go to the movies, hit the gym, or even take a vacation – anything that distracts you from your emotional pain will help you feel better.

Take Up Meditation: Meditation is a great way to deal with emotional stress. In fact, it can help you recover from a variety of stress-related issues. Meditation helps in eliminating emotional tension and diverts your thoughts towards better alternatives. Over time, regular meditation can even improve your focus and boost your self-confidence.

Look for Positivity: Oftentimes, being surrounded by the wrong company or being in a negative environment can contribute to emotional stress, rather than help you manage it. The environment in which you live has a great deal of influence over your personal stress levels, so living in a positive environment is paramount. When dealing with emotional stress, it's imperative that you immerse yourself in a positive environment and surround yourself with people who bring positivity in your life and make you feel good. Depressing and pessimistic people can only add to your pain – avoid interacting with negative people as much as possible.

Diet and Exercise: Something as simple as a balanced diet can also contribute to reducing stress levels. At the very least, don't skip meals. While it's understandable that food would be one of the last things on your mind during a stressful time, an empty stomach can never make you feel good. It's also worth remembering that a fit body means a fit mind. Studies have shown that regular, light to moderate exercise helps keep stress levels low.

Seek Professional Guidance: If you feel that it might help, consider visiting a professional therapist or counselor. Many times, if you feel like you're overwhelmed or that things are only getting worse, a professionally trained therapist or counselor can help you find and overcome the root cause of all your stress.

Emotional stress, regardless of the cause, is something that almost everyone faces at some point in their life. Following the above tips can help you cope with and overcome emotional stress, but ultimately, it's you who's in control of your own life and it's up to you to take those first steps toward a new, stress-free life.

Everyone feels stressed at some point. Occasionally, you may feel a higher level of stress than is common for you. Anxiety or a depressive mood related to high levels of emotional stress are actually quite normal.

What sets standard levels of stress apart from harmful levels is the way they affect your daily life and the methods you use to cope with them.

By clearly identifying the ways in which you exhibit emotional stress and using techniques to cope with the sources (work, school, relationships, etc.), you can deal with the emotional stress present in your life.

Chapter 6:Identifying of Emotional Stressors

1.Look for physical stressors. Stress can be incredibly disruptive to your physical health, as well as your emotional health. In fact, stress places physiological demands on your body that are called an "allostatic load." When this load is too heavy, it can place you at risk for a variety of medical ailments, including serious diseases like diabetes, depression, heart disease, and autoimmune disorders.This is part of why it's so important to keep an eye on your stress levels; it could be causing physical symptoms that you can't otherwise explain and could be damaging your health. Common physical effects of stress can include:

- Headache
- Muscle tension, aches and pains
- Chest pain
- Fatigue or exhaustion
- Alteration of your appetite or sex drive
- Upset stomach and nausea
- Trouble sleeping
- Heartburn or acid reflux

- Difficulty with your bowels

Long-term effects of chronic stress include a weakened immune system, premature aging, increased risk of illness, hypertension, obesity, diabetes, depression, cognitive impairment, inflammatory and autoimmune disorders, heart disease, and greater likelihood of developing illnesses in older age.

2.Examine your recent temper. An overload of stress can manifest itself through a short temper or uncharacteristic difficulty managing anger. Anger (or extreme irritability) is one of the three primary stress emotions, along with anxiety and depression. This symptom of emotional distress is unhealthy for both you and those around you. These changes can also exhibit rapid changes to your mood—or mood swings—due to circumstances that wouldn't typically bother you.

3.Log your sleep patterns. While certain symptoms of emotional stress are easily recognizable, others may be less so. Ongoing sleep disturbances are an indication of stress. You may be sleeping more or less than usual or having trouble falling or staying asleep when you try. If you have trouble sleeping more than one or two nights a week with no identifiable physical reason that your doctor can determine, then emotional stress is a likely candidate.

Chronic tiredness and lethargy are just as often signs of emotional stressors as an inability to sleep, especially if no other illness explains your fatigue.

4.Note changes in your weight or eating habits. If you find yourself eating more than usual or—alternatively—unable to maintain an appetite, this is a common sign of emotional distress. You may also notice fluctuations in weight without any big changes to your diet or exercise routine.

5.Log patterns of obsessive or compulsive behavior. The anxiety associated with emotional distress can find an outlet in obsessive behaviors related to other things. This can range from feeling a compulsion to wash your hands more often than normal all the way to a constant dread that something bad is going to happen.

6.Note the quality of your interactions with others. Another common sign of emotional stress is a change in your social behaviors. This can include anything from staying in far more often (when you used to be more social) to noticing a decline in your sex life with your partner. As with most of these symptoms, you may want to consult your doctor to rule out a potential physical ailment.

You may also see this manifest as a decline in your work or school performance or with colleagues.

7.Look for signs of depression. Chronic stress, or the consistent, grinding stress that lasts for an extended period, has been linked to the development of depression. Studies have shown that stress can shrink the hippocampus, an area of the brain that affects short-term memory, learning, and emotional regulation.This can cause symptoms of depression, which include many of the symptoms mentioned in this article, such as trouble sleeping, change in appetite, and mood disruption. Depression is a serious health condition that often gets worse if left untreated, but it is also highly treatable.You should talk with a healthcare professional if you display these or other symptoms of depression, which include.
Persistent feelings of sadness, emptiness, or anxiety
Feeling hopeless, worthless, or helpless
Loss of interest in things you used to enjoy
Fatigue or exhaustion
Trouble concentrating or making decisions
Changes in appetite, weight, or sleep
Restlessness or irritability
Unexplained physical symptoms
Thoughts of harm, death, or suicide. If you are experiencing any thoughts of harm to yourself or others, call your emergency services or call or text the Suicide and Crisis Lifeline at 988 immediately.
Image titled Deal with Emotional Stress Step 8
8

Determine your level of functioning. Stress is a natural part of human life, and minor stress is often unavoidable. You may have a few areas of dysfunction, such as trouble sleeping or irritability, but not feel unable to cope. However, if you feel that your stress is interfering with your ability to live your life or even get through the day, you should seek help from a health care professional immediately. Here are some signs that your functioning may be impaired and that you should seek help:

You have seen a marked decline in your work or school performance

You feel anxious or depressed

You have begun to use alcohol or drugs to cope

You feel unable to cope, even with everyday things

You are experiencing fears that you can't explain

You have become obsessed with something, such as your weight

You have physical symptoms that your doctor cannot explain

You have withdrawn from people and activities you love

You have thoughts of harm to yourself or others

9.Take a mood test. It can be difficult to determine what you're feeling and whether you should be worried about it. The best option is usually to consult with someone about your thoughts and feelings, but you can also try amood assessment. You can find a self-test at the British National Health Service website here.

These types of self-assessment should not be a replacement for consulting your doctor, but they can help you identify whether your stress is minor and transitory, or whether you have a more serious cause for concern.

Method 2
Coping with Emotional Stress

1.Identify the source of your emotional stress. Emotional stress is akin to the feeling of being on your "last straw" or "last nerve" for an extended period of time.[24] This feeling can present in the varieties of different ways discussed elsewhere in this article. The first step to coping with emotional stress is identifying the source of the stress.

Our work and/or school responsibilities and interpersonal relationships are some of the most common sources of taxing emotional states.

Try writing down things that you feel stressed about. Rank them from 0 (no stress) to 3 (serious stress).

If you have a lot of sources of stress but they're ranked fairly low, or only one or two areas of highly ranked stress, your stress may feel more manageable on your own. If you have many sources of stress that are ranked highly, you should consider seeking professional help, as coping with extreme levels of stress can be very challenging on your own.

2.Accept what you cannot change. It can be very challenging to accept that bad things are happening. However, this simple shift relieves you of the pressure of feeling as if things should be different when they are not.This can apply to anything from the weather to someone's behavior. Obviously, some things are easier to accept than others, but for whatever you cannot control, try to adopt an attitude of acceptance.

3.Practice mindfulness. Mindfulness has been shown to help lower stress and anxiety levels. Mindfulness can expand the hippocampus, the same area shrunk by stress and depression. It can also help rewire your brain's fear responses, resulting in less stress.Mindfulness has even been shown to help battle the effects of depression.

Here are two mindfulness exercises to help you get started.
The "finding silver linings" exercise. This exercise has been shown to reduce depressive symptoms and can help you build resilience to stress.

Begin by listing 5 things that make you happy or that you value.
Focus on a source of stress for you right now. Write down a few sentences about the situation and how it

made you feel. Try to show yourself compassion as you write, not judging yourself for your feelings. For example: "I'm feeling stressed because my partner doesn't talk to me as much anymore."

Now try to find three little "silver linings" to the situation. This step takes a lot of practice and a willingness to be open, but it can help you. For example, "This situation is an opportunity for me to practice acceptance for my partner" or "This situation reminds me how much I value communication." It can be hard to see the bright side, especially of an upsetting situation, but give it a go. Try this for 10 minutes a day for 3 weeks.

The "self-compassion break." We are sometimes a source of our own stress, particularly if we're judging ourselves for perceived mistakes or failings. Learning to take a quick 5-minute self-compassion break every day can help you break this habit of judging yourself harshly, which can help reduce your stress levels.

Begin by selecting a situation that is causing you stress, such as "I'm afraid that I'm not a good mother to my son because I have to work so much.

Notice how the stress feels in your body when you think about this situation. What sensations do you experience? You might experience a rapid heartbeat, a fluttery stomach, nausea, etc.

Say gently to yourself, "This is a moment of stress." It's important to acknowledge when we're in pain, rather than try to ignore or repress it.

Remind yourself, "Stress is something everyone struggles with." It can help to remind yourself of your common humanity: you aren't alone, and it is natural to experience stress in our lives.

Place your hands over your heart, or wrap your arms around your body to give yourself a hug. Gently say, "May I show myself kindness" or "May I accept myself."

You can say any phrase that seems meaningful to you, as long as it is compassionate and positive.

Repeat this at least once a day, but you can do it whenever you're having a moment of stress.

4.Identify a support system. The trusted ear of a family member, friend, or even a mental health professional can help you feel better when you express your emotions about stress.

Sometimes these individuals can offer potentially valuable feedback. Even a sympathetic and caring presence will ensure that you do not feel alone with your stress.

A study with cancer patients found that the greater amount of social support a patient reported, the less they reported mood disturbance.

It is important that your support system is constituted of people who will truly support you. Find those who will listen to your concerns and fears without being judgmental, angry, or trying to "fix" something that cannot be changed.

5.Exercise regularly. Emotional stress often feels like a lack of control over your life, and maintaining an exercise routine is a great way to take back some of that control. Exercising also provides an outlet for some of the stressful energy, and it helps the body produce pleasurable endorphins when you feel accomplished after a good workout. Though fatigue may be one of your stress symptoms, you should still try your hardest to exercise regularly.

A heightened amount of physical activity may also help with stress-related sleep disturbances if you're experiencing them as part of your symptoms.

6.Solve smaller problems. Another great way to help yourself feel like you're regaining control is to focus on a number of smaller problems you're confronting.This allows you to shift your focus from larger issues while also finding resolutions to smaller ones. You may even begin feeling like the larger problems are more manageable with some smaller ones behind you.
This also means setting realistic goals at work, school, and home. You can't mitigate stress while still overloading yourself with it.

Setting smaller, realistic goals can mean tackling a specific homework assignment at school as opposed to worrying about your grade for the entire semester.
At work, you might set a daily to-do list for certain parts of a project rather than allowing the entire project to daunt you.

7.Eat a well-balanced diet. Though you may find it difficult if a lack of appetite is one of your symptoms, a well-balanced diet is always a crucial part of feeling physically and mentally healthy. If fatigue and lethargy are some of your stress symptoms, then eating better will help provide you with daily energy as well.

8.Participate in things you enjoy. Even while emotionally stressed, we all still take joy in hobbies, crafts, or other personal activities. Try to make more time for the things that make you happy.This can be anything from sports with friends to spending time with a great book.
If you can't think of a single activity to fit this step, then your stressful situation may have developed into an actual depression. In this case, your physician or a mental health professional may be able to help.

9.Change your environment. Many of the things leading to your emotional distress may stem from the things you encounter on a daily basis. If the daily news stresses you out or the same commute to work every day, then try changing those things in your daily environment. Isolate and avoid as many of these daily stressors as you can and try your hardest to accept that you cannot change the others.

10. Keep a stress journal. Emotional stress doesn't always occur when your support network is available to listen. A stress journal gives you a chance to write down the source of your stress and exactly how it made you feel, which is a great alternative to venting those feelings to a friend or family member.

This approach even allows you to write down how you feel you handled the stress, which can help you discover your own best practices for coping.

For instance, you may realize once you go to write it down that a discussion with a significant other turned into an argument around a certain topic. You can use that information to think closely about the topic and a better way to handle the discussion next time it arises.

Work to resolve interpersonal conflicts. Ongoing conflicts with those close to you are some of the prime sources of emotional stress. Working to resolve these conflicts wherever possible is a huge step toward mitigating emotional distress.

When dealing with potentially tense interactions during these conflicts, express your feelings assertively without letting the person take advantage of you, but always do so respectfully as well.

Remember that negotiation and compromise is the best way to defuse interpersonal conflict in a productive way.

Engage in meditation or prayer. Meditation is a form of guided thought wherein you focus typically on one specific action, such as breathing (or stretching in the case of yoga). If you are spiritual or religious, you may find a similar form of calm and peace in prayer.

Deep, relaxed breathing by itself is a great way to combat stress..

Relaxation training is another form of meditation. Find a quiet, comfortable position and flex each muscle in your body one muscle group at a time. Start with your toes and work your way up.

Method 3

Finding Professional Help to Deal with Emotional Stress

1.See your doctor. Your plain old physician can be the best place to start when seeking professional help for emotional stress. You may have several physical symptoms in addition to emotional ones associated with your stress, and your doctor will help diagnose the symptoms.

Based on the symptoms, your doctor will also be able to help you decide whether you should see a counselor/psychologist or a psychiatrist.

As actual doctors, psychiatrists can prescribe medication, and much of the treatment may deal with medication management. Licensed psychologists and counselors, on the other hand, have PhDs and MAs (respectively), but they are not MDs and cannot prescribe medication.

Psychologists and counselors will use a variety of therapeutic tools aimed at helping you change the behaviors or ways of thinking that lead to your stressful reactions to situations. Psychologists are more likely to do academic research in the field of psychology in addition to working with patients as well. You won't necessarily receive a better form of care from one or the other. The key is to find a licensed professional who listens and with whom you feel comfortable sharing your emotional stressors.

Some instances, such as those dealing with depression or anxiety, may call for both a psychiatrist to manage medications and a psychologist or counselor from whom you can learn other coping techniques.

Image titled Deal with Emotional Stress Step

2.Learn therapeutic techniques. If you and your doctor don't feel your situation warrants medication, a licensed psychologist or counselor can help you find other techniques for dealing with emotional stress in addition to being great listeners. Cognitive-behavioral therapy (CBT) is one example of a technique to help cope with emotional stress and the related anxiety.

With CBT, the therapist helps you become highly aware of your own patterns of thinking and behavior with the goal of helping you to avoid the emotional stress involved with those common patterns.

Even if your doctor decides that your situation warrants a medication prescription, you should still consider seeing a therapist as well. Medicating the problem can help you to manage the symptoms, but it won't assist you in dealing with the root causes of the stress.

Image titled Deal with Emotional Stress Step 24

3.See a psychiatrist. Emotional stress can easily lead to too much depression or anxiety for a person to manage on his or her own, and this can occasionally mean the use of mood-altering medications while dealing with the worst parts of an emotionally stressful situation. A wide array of drugs are available and meeting with a psychiatrist will help him or her prescribe the drug best suited for your situation.

Commonly prescribed medications in these situations include: selective serotonin reuptake inhibitors (SSRIs) such as Celexa, Lexapro, Paxil, Prozac, and Zoloft; selective serotonin and norepinephrine inhibitors (SNRIs) such as Cymbalta and Effexor; and monoamine oxidase inhibitors (MAOIs) such as Nardil and Parnate. Your psychiatrist may prescribe any of the above for symptoms of depression, whereas SSRIs specifically have proven effective for treating anxiety disorders.

Most mental health professionals will suggest the use of a medication in combination with the other steps here. Relying on medication alone is far from the most effective way to deal with an emotionally stressful life event.

Always take the medication exactly as prescribed, and consult with your psychiatrist before stopping usage.

Image titled Deal with Emotional Stress Step.

Follow up with the care professional regularly. Many people quickly feel discouraged with the therapy or counseling process due to the lack of immediate results. Talking through your emotionally stressful issues, learning techniques to handle them, and normalizing those techniques as part of your standard reaction to stress will not be a quick process. Have patience with the treatment and keep up with your appointments for as long as your therapist suggests in order to reap worthwhile results from the process.

References
Springer link
https://link.springer.com/referenceworkentry/10.1007/97
8-1-4419-1005-9_289
Emotional Stress: Warning Signs, Management, When to
Get Help
https://my.clevelandclinic.org/health/articles/6406-emoti
onal-stress-warning-signs-management-when-to-get-help
6 Signs of Emotional Stress and How to Overcome it
https://reallifecounseling.us/signs-of-emotional-stress/
Ways to Cope With Emotional Stress
https://www.verywellmind.com/coping-with-emotional-s
tress-3144565
Stress Symptoms
https://www.webmd.com/balance/stress-management/str
ess-symptoms-effects_of-stress-on-the-body